MAJOR INCIDENT MANAGEMENT SYSTEM

The scene aide memoire for
MAJOR INCIDENT MEDICAL
MANAGEMENT AND SUPPORT

➤ **Timothy J Hodgetts**

Defence Consultant Adviser, Emergency Medicine
Honorary Professor, Emergency Medicine & Trauma

➤ **Crispin Porter**

Specialist Registrar, Emergency Medicine

BMJ
Books

©BMJ Books 2002

BMJ Books is an imprint of the BMJ Publishing Group

First published in 2002
9 2012
BMJ Books, BMA House, Tavistock Square, London WC1H 9JR

This book is the second edition of *The Pre-Hospital Emergency Management Master* published in 1995.

This book supports the popular *Major Incident Medical Management and Support* ("MIMMS") course that provides the only international standard for medical management at the scene of a multiple casualty incident. Like the second edition of MIMMS (2002), this book is generic in its approach with principles that cross international and civilian-military boundaries.

British Library Cataloguing in Publication Data

A catalogue record for this book is available from the British Library

ISBN 13: 978-0-7279-1614-3

Printed and bound in Singapore by Ho Printing Singapore Pte Ltd

Contents

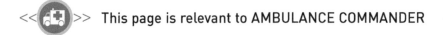

Symbol Key

<< 🚑 >>   This page is relevant to AMBULANCE COMMANDER

<< DOC >>   This page is relevant to MEDICAL COMMANDER

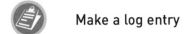   Make a log entry

📱   Send a message

👫   Talk face-to-face

<< ◇X◇ >>   Go to page indicated

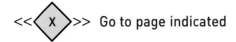

Terminology

This pocket aide memoire uses the generic terminology
adopted by the international Major Incident Medical
Management and Support system. For example, the term
'AMBULANCE COMMANDER' describes the role of the
officer responsible for all ambulance assets at the scene,
although it is recognised that other terminology may be
used in individual countries.

FIRST
ACTIONS

first ambulance at scene

first doctor at scene

first ambulance at scene

➤ Start a log and record time of arrival

➤ Wear protective clothing
  - helmet
  - high visibility coat or tabard

➤ Make METHANE assessment and send METHANE report

➤ Consider where arriving ambulances should park

➤ Consider where casualty clearing station should be placed
  - safe distance from incident (discuss with FIRE)
  - on vehicle circuit (discuss with POLICE)
  - on hard standing where possible
  - using available shelter

➤ Consider place for helicopter landing site (discuss with POLICE) and ensure this is marked

➤ Continue to assess and communicate with AMBULANCE CONTROL as details become available

➤ Continue duties of SILVER AMBULANCE COMMANDER until relieved

1

first doctor at scene

➤ Start a log and record time of arrival

➤ Wear protective clothing
  - helmet
  - high visibility coat or tabard

➤ Liaise with SILVER AMBULANCE COMMANDER and record his/her name

➤ Receive and record METHANE brief

➤ Obtain
  - radio, where issued
  - spare battery
  - headset or earpiece
  - call-sign for yourself and ambulance commander
  - tabard (vest) for medical commander

➤ Assume duties of SILVER MEDICAL COMMANDER until relieved

11

METHANE report

METHANE report

CHALET report

METHANE report

M My call-sign, or name and appointment
Major incident STANDBY or DECLARED

E Exact location
- grid reference, or GPS where available

T Type of incident

H Hazards, present and potential

A Access to scene, and egress route
- helicopter landing site location

N Number and severity of casualties

E Emergency services, present and required

CHALET report

C   Casualties, number and severity

H   Hazards, present and potential

A   Access to scene, and egress route
- helicopter landing site location

L   Location, exact
- grid reference, or GPS where available

E   Emergency services, present and required

T   Type of incident

> Some emergency services use CHALET.
> METHANE is CHALET in a logical order

COMMAND

3

tiers of command

precedence at the scene

scene organisation

personnel recognition

hierarchy of ambulance command

hierarchy of medical command

briefing for duty

tiers of command

BRONZE
➤ The BRONZE area is the area of immediate hazard and casualty rescue
➤ The boundary of the BRONZE area is the INNER CORDON
➤ Each service may designate a BRONZE COMMANDER
➤ There can be more than one BRONZE area (and set of bronze commanders) within an incident

SILVER
➤ The SILVER area is the entire scene
➤ The boundary of the SILVER area is the OUTER CORDON
➤ Each service will provide a SILVER COMMANDER
➤ There is only one SILVER area for an incident (exception is an incident over a wide area, for example an earthquake, with multiple "major incidents")

GOLD
➤ GOLD represents the highest level of command for the incident
➤ GOLD is remote from the scene
➤ GOLD may be identified by a local authority, regional, county, state or national boundary

tiers of command

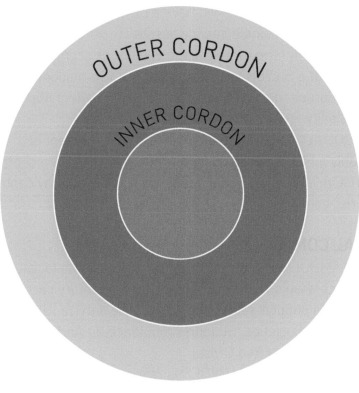

■ BRONZE

■ SILVER

■ GOLD

precedence at the scene

SCENE CONTROL

➤ Each service at the scene will have a COMMANDER, who is responsible for all single service assets

➤ One service will have overall responsibility, or scene CONTROL

➤ CONTROL at a SILVER level in UK is a POLICE responsibility. In other European countries (Netherlands, Sweden) it is a FIRE responsibility

➤ CONTROL at a BRONZE level when hazard is present is invariably a FIRE responsibility (an exception may be a chemical terrorist incident where specialist trained POLICE may control the inner cordon)

MEDICAL COMMAND

➤ SILVER AMBULANCE COMMANDER is responsible for all ambulance assets at the scene, including voluntary personnel working in a support role to the ambulance service (UK Voluntary Aid Societies: St John Ambulance, St Andrew Ambulance, British Red Cross)

➤ SILVER MEDICAL COMMANDER is responsible for all doctors and nurses at the scene

➤ Precedence must be established before there is a difference of opinion between health service SILVER COMMANDERS. This is not formalised in UK (but, for example, in Australia it is formally the MEDICAL COMMANDER)

SCENE ORGANISATION

OFF SCENE MARSHALLING AREA

MEDIA LIAISON POINT

INCIDENT CONTROL POINT

outer cordon

inner cordon

AMBULANCE PARKING POINT

AMBULANCE LOADING POINT

CASUALTY CLEARING STATION

SURVIVOR RECEPTION CENTRE

PATIENTS

SURVIVORS

INCIDENT

JOINT SERVICES EMERGENCY CONTROL

personnel recognition

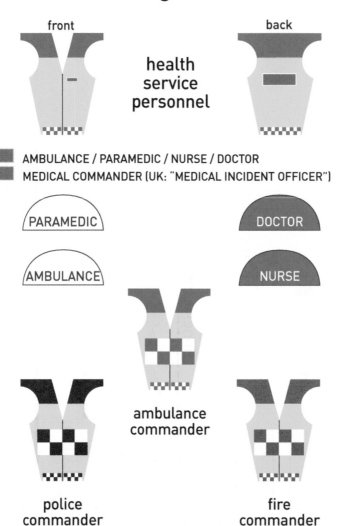

front

back

health service personnel

AMBULANCE / PARAMEDIC / NURSE / DOCTOR
MEDICAL COMMANDER (UK: "MEDICAL INCIDENT OFFICER")

PARAMEDIC

DOCTOR

AMBULANCE

NURSE

ambulance commander

police commander

fire commander

hierarchy of ambulance command

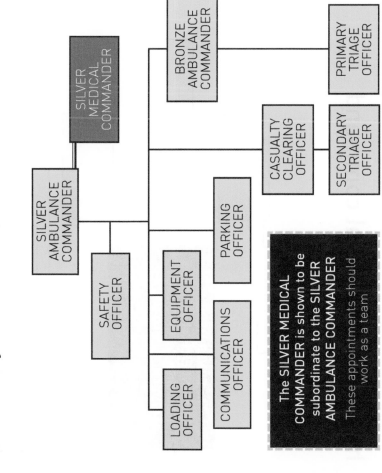

SILVER MEDICAL COMMANDER

SILVER AMBULANCE COMMANDER

BRONZE AMBULANCE COMMANDER

PRIMARY TRIAGE OFFICER

CASUALTY CLEARING OFFICER

SECONDARY TRIAGE OFFICER

SAFETY OFFICER

EQUIPMENT OFFICER

PARKING OFFICER

LOADING OFFICER

COMMUNICATIONS OFFICER

The SILVER MEDICAL COMMANDER is shown to be subordinate to the SILVER AMBULANCE COMMANDER

These appointments should work as a team

<< DOC >>

hierarchy of medical command

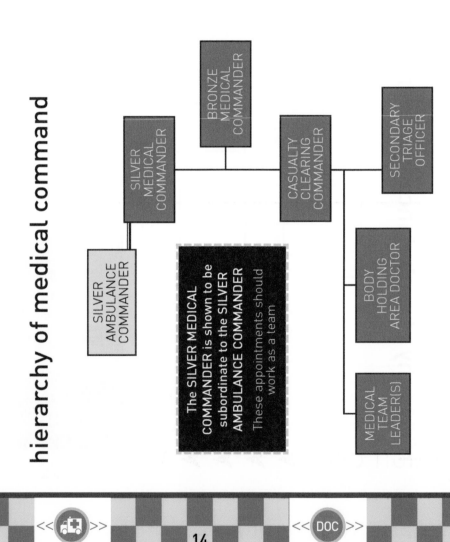

SILVER AMBULANCE COMMANDER

SILVER MEDICAL COMMANDER

BRONZE MEDICAL COMMANDER

The SILVER MEDICAL COMMANDER is shown to be subordinate to the SILVER AMBULANCE COMMANDER

These appointments should work as a team

CASUALTY CLEARING COMMANDER

MEDICAL TEAM LEADER(S)

BODY HOLDING AREA DOCTOR

SECONDARY TRIAGE OFFICER

<< DOC >>

briefing for duty (1)

Commanders must brief all key personnel. Write a briefing in your LOG to include the following:

➤ Introduction
- Introduce yourself and establish who are the personnel present at the briefing

➤ Situation
- Give a brief description of the:
  - type of incident
  - time of the incident and subsequent response
  - the estimated total number of casualties
  - the estimated number of casualties remaining on the scene
- State the size of the medical response:
  - number of ambulance personnel
  - number of immediate care doctors
  - number of hospital teams

➤ Geography
- Describe the incident site including:
  - the boundaries of the BRONZE and SILVER areas
  - any important features (access routes, railways, pylons, obstacles, hazards)
  - the grid reference (if maps available)

➤ Aim
- State the aim of the medical services at the incident and repeat this for clarity

➤ Individual tasks
- Address each key person or team and give an individual task briefing **(hand out action cards)**

briefing for duty (2)

➤ Command and control
- All personnel are responsible to the SILVER COMMANDER (ambulance or medical), therefore:
  - all tasks must be authorised by the SILVER COMMANDER
  - any new staff must be sent to the SILVER COMMANDER for tasking

➤ Communications
- Clearly indicate the location of the SILVER ambulance control vehicle
- Confirm the the following radio call-signs:
  - the SILVER AMBULANCE CONTROL VEHICLE
  - SILVER / BRONZE COMMANDERS
  - all other key personnel issued radios
- State the importance of non-radio communication (face-to-face, runners)

➤ Logistics and support
- Confirm what equipment individuals have brought, and what else is available
- Confirm resupply is through CCS COMMANDER (CCS personnel) or BRONZE COMMANDER (forward personnel)
- State where food and drink is available, and when staff can expect to be relieved

➤ Timings
- Give the time and place of the next meeting, if appropriate

**Move around the group and give individuals
the opportunity to ask questions**

SAFETY

4

safety

SAFETY PRIORITIES
➤ The following safety priorities should be observed:
- **Self**
- **Scene**
- **Survivors (injured and uninjured)**

PERSONAL SAFETY
➤ Appropriate protective equipment is essential:
- high visibility jacket or tabard (vest)
- protective boots
- hard hat
- goggles or visor
- ear defenders
- gloves (heavy duty and latex)

➤ **DO NOT** approach the incident when hazards are known to exist without permission of the BRONZE FIRE COMMANDER (direct permission, or indirectly through BRONZE AMBULANCE COMMANDER)

SCENE SAFETY

➤ Safety inside the BRONZE area is the responsibility of the BRONZE FIRE COMMANDER. When there is fire or toxic chemicals the BRONZE FIRE COMMANDER will take CONTROL of the BRONZE AREA. Safety inside the SILVER area is a responsibility of the POLICE who will evacuate any population at risk

➤ If first on the scene, the AMBULANCE COMMANDER will take CONTROL until additional resources arrive, and will:
  - Assume that hazards (actual or potential) exist
  - Remember the **THREE** Cs of immediate incident CONTROL:
    - CONFIRM the nature of the incident and any hazards
    - CLEAR the area of bystanders and walking casualties
    - CORDON the area to prevent further casualties

SURVIVOR SAFETY

➤ Occasionally it will be necessary to move casualties if there is an immediate threat to life such as fire or toxic chemicals. This will be done *without* the usual precautions employed during controlled extrication (e.g. spinal immobilisation)

➤ Measures must be taken to avoid additional casualties by preventing hypothermia, heat illness, exhaustion and dehydration

HAZCHEM recognition

➤ The recognition and neutralising of hazardous chemicals is a responsibility of the FIRE SERVICE
➤ A board displaying details of the hazardous chemical is required on all vehicles in which they are transported

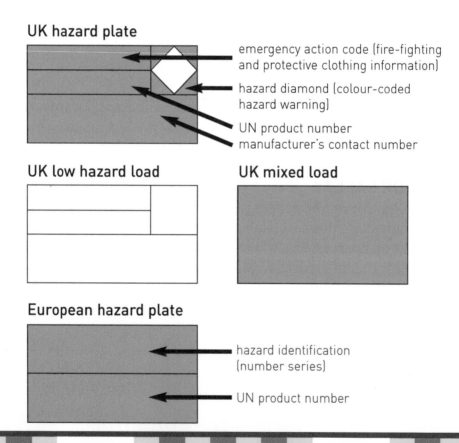

UK hazard plate

emergency action code (fire-fighting and protective clothing information)

hazard diamond (colour-coded hazard warning)

UN product number
manufacturer's contact number

UK low hazard load

UK mixed load

European hazard plate

hazard identification (number series)

UN product number

decontamination

Casualty decontamination is a responsibility of the HEALTH SERVICES

The following procedure applies to decontamination from hazardous chemical, radiation or bio-hazard.

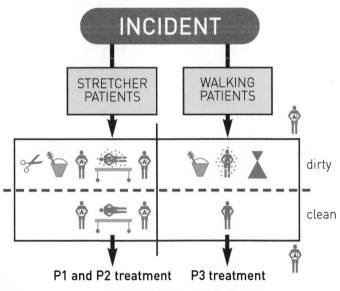

dirty

clean

P1 and P2 treatment   P3 treatment

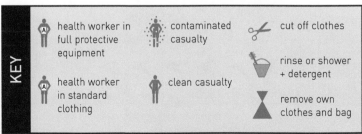

KEY

health worker in full protective equipment	contaminated casualty	cut off clothes
health worker in standard clothing	clean casualty	rinse or shower + detergent
		remove own clothes and bag

COMMUNICATIONS

5

using a radio

IF YOU ARE ISSUED A RADIO IT MUST BE MONITORED AT ALL TIMES: OTHERWISE IT MAY BE PRESUMED YOU HAVE HEARD A GROUP MESSAGE

CHECK LIST
➤ Ask for a spare battery
➤ Ask for a headset or ear-piece (if available)
➤ Ask for YOUR call-sign and other key call-signs
➤ Ask how the radio is turned on/off, and the volume adjusted
➤ Ask how the battery is removed

TO TRANSMIT
➤ Hold the radio a few centimetres in front of your mouth.
➤ Do NOT hold the radio like a telephone: you may be talking into the battery and will not be heard
➤ Hold down the long button on the side of the radio (PRESS-TO-TALK switch)
➤ Talk slowly, and for no more than 20–30 seconds before asking for acknowledgement
➤ Release the PRESS-TO-TALK switch to receive

TO CHANGE THE BATTERY
➤ Turn the radio OFF
➤ Engage the battery release switch
➤ Remove the dead battery
➤ Replace with a fresh battery
➤ Turn the radio ON and perform a radio check

key words

Key words are used to ensure **ACCURACY** and **BREVITY** of radio messages:

OVER	I have finished talking and I want the other call-sign to respond
OUT	I have finished talking and the communication is terminated
OK	I understand
ROGER	I understand and will comply with request
SAY AGAIN	Repeat your message [all after... / all before... / from... to...]
ACKNOWLEDGE	I need confirmation you have received important information (may reply 'OK', 'ROGER' or by repeating key information)
SPELL	Precedes important word being spelled using phonetic alphabet, for example, "I need entonox, SPELL echo-november-tango etc..."
FIGURES	Precedes long number being spoken digit by digit, for example, "one hundred, FIGURES one-zero-zero"
WRONG	I have made a mistake, for example, "there are six dead, WRONG seven dead"

phonetic alphabet

alpha	juliet	sierra
bravo	kilo	tango
charlie	lima	uniform
delta	mike	victor
echo	november	whiskey
foxtrot	oscar	x-ray
golf	papa	yankee
hotel	quebec	zulu
india	romeo	

alternative methods

FACE-TO-FACE	Essential for commanders
	Briefings every 15–30mins at start
RUNNER	Send a WRITTEN message
	Consider volunteer personnel
MEGAPHONE	Useful for group messages
	Beware of overuse: less effective
WHISTLE	Generally reserved to indicate escalation
	of threat and need to evacuate
HAND SIGNALS	Useful to communicate over large distance
	when voice cannot be heard
	Need line of sight
	Must be taught to understand signals
PAGER	Useful for group messages
	Vibrate mode may be more effective when
	high background noise
MOBILE PHONE	Effective 1-to-1 communication
	No need for radio voice procedure
	Poor control of medical messages
	System can be overloaded

common hand signals

Hand signals are useful to communicate over a large distance when voice cannot be heard. Direct line of sight is required. Those to whom the signals are directed must be taught to understand them.

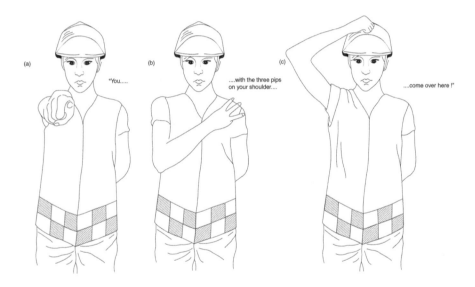

(a)

"You....."

(b)

....with the three pips on your shoulder....

(c)

....come over here !"

dealing with the media

ALL MAJOR INCIDENTS WILL ATTRACT A SUBSTANTIAL MEDIA RESPONSE: THE SILVER POLICE COMMANDER IS RESPONSIBLE FOR MANAGING THE MEDIA

GENERAL APPROACH
➤ Prepare a statement in advance if possible
➤ Anticipate what questions will be asked:
- What happened? What are you doing? How many casualties?

DO NOT be drawn into suppositions regarding the cause and responsibility for the incident

BEFORE A TELEVISION INTERVIEW
➤ Check your appearance: do you look professional?
➤ Be clear on your key messages (up to three recommended)
➤ Ask what the first question will be
➤ Find out the "wind up" signal, so you will not be cut off mid-sentence

DURING A TELEVISION INTERVIEW
➤ Always assume that you are on the air
➤ STAND STILL: look straight at the interviewer, not the camera
➤ **A**nswer the question, **B**ridge the gap to your key message(s) and **C**ommunicate your key message(s)

Prepare media statement notes in your log

TRIAGE

triage sieve
triage sort
use of expectant category
paediatric triage

6

triage sieve

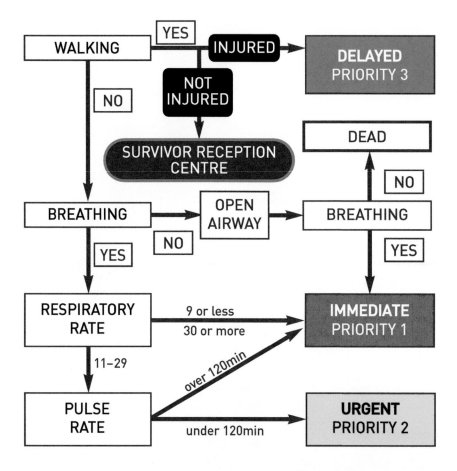

Capillary refill test (CRT) is an alternative to pulse rate, but is unreliable in the cold or dark: if it is used, a CRT of >2 seconds indicates PRIORITY 1

triage sort

STEP 1: Calculate the GLASGOW COMA SCORE (GCS)

A Eye opening:		B Verbal response:		C Motor response:	
spontaneous	4	orientated	5	obeys commands	6
to voice	3	confused	4	localises	5
to pain	2	inappropriate	3	pain withdraws	4
none	1	incomprehensible	2	pain flexes	3
		no response	1	pain extends	2
				no response	1

GCS= A + B + C

STEP 2: calculate the TRIAGE SORT SCORE

X GCS		Y Respiratory rate		Z Systolic BP	
13–15	4	10–29	4	≥90	4
9–12	3	≥30	3	76–89	3
6–8	2	6–9	2	50–75	2
4–5	1	1–5	1	1–49	1
3	0	0	0	0	0

TRIAGE SORT SCORE = X + Y + Z

STEP 3: Assign a triage PRIORITY

> **12 = PRIORITY 3**
> 11 = PRIORITY 2
> ≤10 = PRIORITY 1

STEP 4: Upgrade PRIORITY at discretion of senior clinician, dependent on the anatomical injury/working diagnosis

expectant category

➤ The EXPECTANT category represents patients who will die even if they receive optimal treatment

➤ This category is used only if medical resources are OVERWHELMED, and may be revoked when adequate resources become available: in the event of improved resources, EXPECTANT patients are recategorised as PRIORITY 1

➤ EXPECTANT patients may be identified in a variety of ways:

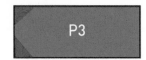

with a blue triage label

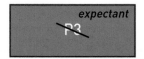

with a green label endorsed 'EXPECTANT'

P3

or with the corners of a green label folded back over red

paediatric triage: principles

➤ The adult triage systems may be applied to children but:
  - The physiological differences between adults and children might result in a disproportionate number of children being triaged IMMEDIATE, PRIORITY 1
  - There can be difficulties with applying the adult Glasgow Coma Scale to infants and young children

An adjusted paediatric triage protocol can be utilised dependent upon the body length (or weight) of the child. The general principles are:

➤ If a child is "alert and moving all limbs" OR walking, they are DELAYED, PRIORITY 3 for treatment/evacuation
➤ If NOT DELAYED, PRIORITY 3, use a paediatric triage protocol dependent upon the body length (or age) of the child
➤ A trapped child is IMMEDIATE, PRIORITY 1 until released, whereupon use a length-related triage protocol
➤ Measure the body length by placing a tape measure alongside the child in a prone position. If not available and the child's age is known, then estimate the body weight using the following formula:

$$2 \times (\text{age in years} + 4) = \text{weight (kg)}$$

➤ If a child is on the boundary between two protocols use the protocol for the larger child

USE ADULT TRIAGE SYSTEMS IF CHILD IS LONGER THAN 140 cm OR HEAVIER THAN 32 kg

paediatric triage protocol – 1

50–80cm (or 3–10kg)

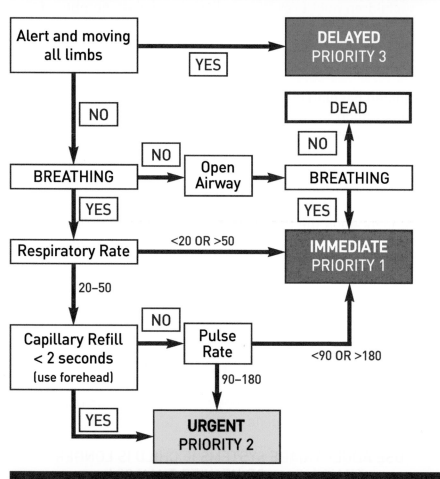

paediatric triage protocol – 2

80–100cm (or 11–18kg)

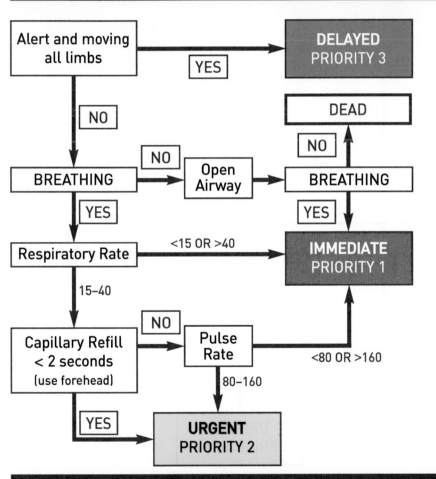

Alert and moving all limbs → YES → **DELAYED** PRIORITY 3

NO

BREATHING → NO → **Open Airway** → **BREATHING** → NO → **DEAD**

BREATHING → YES → **IMMEDIATE** PRIORITY 1

Respiratory Rate → <15 OR >40 → **IMMEDIATE** PRIORITY 1

15–40

Capillary Refill < 2 seconds (use forehead) → NO → **Pulse Rate** → <80 OR >160 → **IMMEDIATE** PRIORITY 1

Pulse Rate → 80–160 → **URGENT** PRIORITY 2

Capillary Refill → YES → **URGENT** PRIORITY 2

SEND UNINJURED SURVIVORS TO SURVIVOR RECEPTION CENTRE

paediatric triage protocol – 3

100–140cm (or 19–32kg)

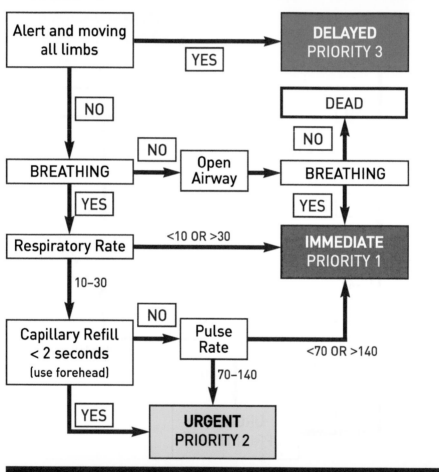

SEND UNINJURED SURVIVORS TO SURVIVOR RECEPTION CENTRE

TREATMENT

treatment priorities
Casualty Clearing Station
(CCS) layout

7

treatment priorities

Treatment priorities for individual patients follow best practice within the constraints of a multiple casualty incident:

AIRWAY, with cervical spine control where appropriate
BREATHING, with oxygen where available
CIRCULATION, with control of external bleeding always

Major incident treatment limitations

➤ Full *spinal immobilisation* is impractical for all victims of, for example, a rail crash, even though they are exposed to the same mechanism of injury. Clinical judgement must be exercised to a greater extent than in a single casualty blunt trauma incident

➤ *Oxygen* is a limited resource: more than one patient can be given oxygen from the same cylinder (use a Y connector), but individual flow rates may be reduced

➤ *Defibrillation* may be appropriate in the casualty clearing station for a witnessed cardiac arrest: those with no vital signs at the site of injury should be pronounced dead

➤ *Intubation* can only be performed by paramedics on unresponsive (dead or nearly dead) patients: it has a limited role at the scene

CCS layout

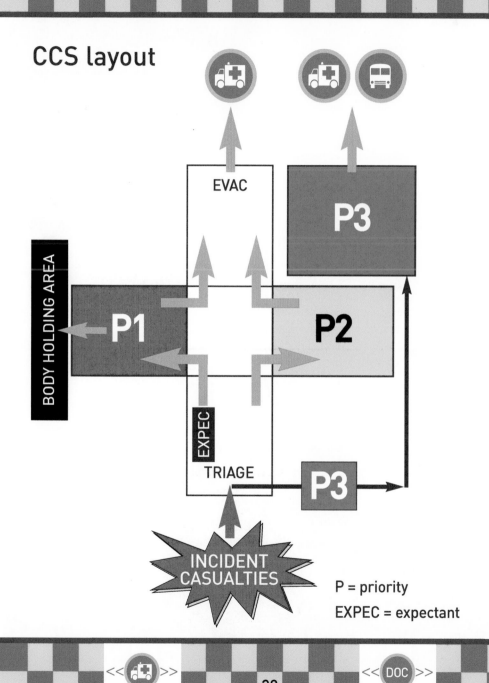

BODY HOLDING AREA

EVAC

P3

P1

P2

EXPEC

TRIAGE

P3

INCIDENT CASUALTIES

P = priority

EXPEC = expectant

<< DOC >>

TRANSPORT

casualty evacuation principles
vehicle selection
helicopter landing site selection
helicopter landing site marking
helicopter marshalling
helicopter loading

8

casualty evacuation principles

➤ There will be a finite number of emergency ambulances available for the evacuation of casualties
➤ The SILVER AMBULANCE COMMANDER and the AMBULANCE LOADING OFFICER are responsible for the efficient use of available transport for patient evacuation

IMMEDIATE PRIORITY 1

➤ These casualties should be evacuated by emergency ambulance:
  • Where appropriate, consider the use of ambulance helicopters
  • Consider the level of escort required (paramedic/nurse/doctor/anaesthetist)

URGENT PRIORITY 2

➤ These casualties might need to be moved by emergency ambulance, but PRIORITY 1 have precedence (P2 may be moved first if P1 packaging is incomplete)

DELAYED PRIORITY 3

➤ These casualties often do not need to be moved by emergency ambulance, unless there are adequate resources for all patients: consider alternative means

SILVER COMMANDERS ARE TO ENSURE THE BEST USE OF TRANSPORT AND APPROPRIATE DISTRIBUTION OF CASUALTIES

vehicle selection

➤ Emergency ambulances are not required for the evacuation of all casualties, especially PRIORITY 3. Consider using alternative modes of transport such as:
- voluntary aid organisation ambulances
- outpatient ambulance vehicles (minibuses)
- bus or coach
- train
- non-ambulance service helicopters

➤ Use of a range of modes of transport will facilitate a wider distribution of casualties

HELICOPTERS
➤ **Advantages**
- fast movement of selected casualties/medical teams
- able to reach geographically remote incidents
- rapid transit to distant specialised hospitals

➤ **Disadvantages**
- limited casualty capacity
- limited availability
- limited capability for in-transit observation and treatment of casualty

landing site: selection

This is the recommended landing site preparation when the exact details of the aircraft are unknown

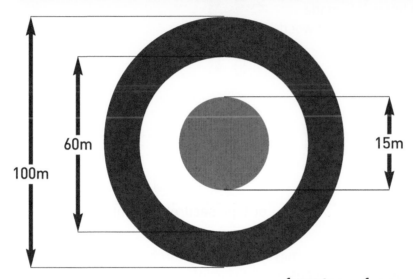

100m

60m

15m

1 metre = 1 pace

All areas must be cleared of loose objects

Ideally ground should be level: if sloping, slope should be uniform and <10°

Hard standing or firm ground capable of taking at least 4 tons

Cleared to ground level

Cleared to 0.6m (2 feet)

helicopter landing site: marking

BY DAY

Use a letter "H" made
from large pieces of wood

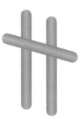

rocks...

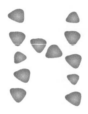

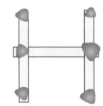

or tape **securely** weighted...

...or use a flashing mirror, a flashing torch light
(vehicle roof beacons will be visible)...

  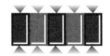

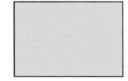

or a fluorescent panel

helicopter landing site: marking

BY NIGHT

Use lights (torches, chemiluminescent light-sticks – but not blue light) of equal intensity to form a letter 'T'...

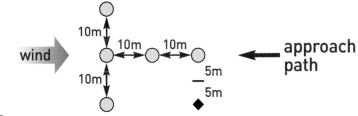

wind

10m
10m 10m
10m
5m
5m

approach
path

○ Light
— Touchdown point
◆ Load point

1 metre = 1 pace

...or use vehicles (cars, not lorries) with beam headlights...

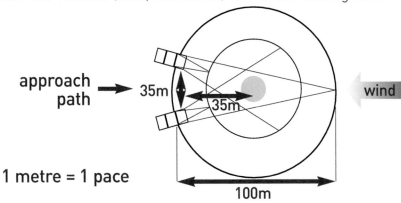

approach
path → 35m

35m

wind

1 metre = 1 pace

100m

THIS IS ONLY TO BE USED AS A SECOND CHOICE

helicopter marshalling (1)

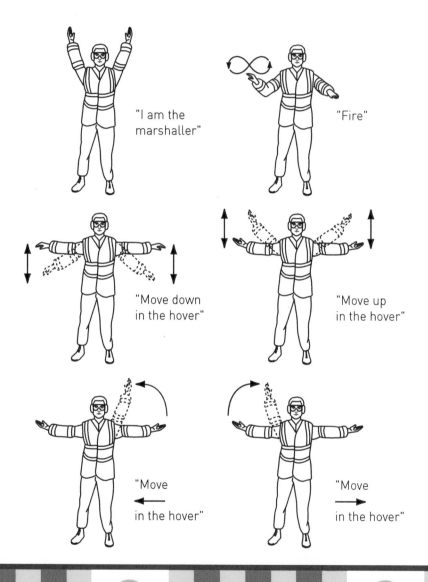

"I am the
marshaller"

"Fire"

"Move down
in the hover"

"Move up
in the hover"

"Move
←
in the hover"

"Move
→
in the hover"

helicopter marshalling (2)

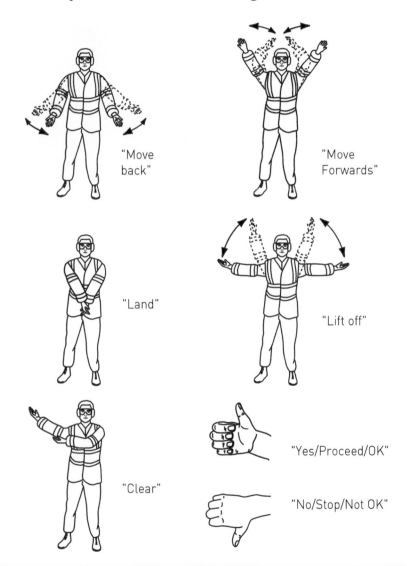

"Move back"

"Move Forwards"

"Land"

"Lift off"

"Clear"

"Yes/Proceed/OK"

"No/Stop/Not OK"

helicopter loading

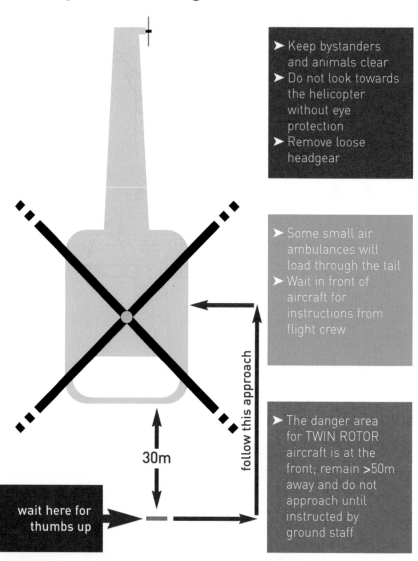

- ➤ Keep bystanders and animals clear
- ➤ Do not look towards the helicopter without eye protection
- ➤ Remove loose headgear

- ➤ Some small air ambulances will load through the tail
- ➤ Wait in front of aircraft for instructions from flight crew

- ➤ The danger area for TWIN ROTOR aircraft is at the front; remain >50m away and do not approach until instructed by ground staff

follow this approach

30m

wait here for thumbs up

<< DOC >>

ACTION CARDS
ambulance personnel

1   silver ambulance commander

2   bronze ambulance commander

3   CCS officer

4   communications officer

5   equipment officer

6   loading officer

7   parking officer

8   primary triage officer

9   safety officer

10   secondary triage officer

1-10

silver ambulance commander

COMMAND
➤ Take COMMAND of all ambulance (including voluntary) assets; make key appointments
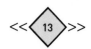

➤ Wear the tabard to identify yourself as the SILVER AMBULANCE COMMANDER and remain near emergency services control vehicles as much as possible
➤ Start a log of your actions, noting the time for each entry; use a scribe when available

SAFETY
➤ Take responsibility for the safety of all health service personnel at scene, or delegate this to SAFETY OFFICER (action card 9)

COMMUNICATIONS
➤ LIAISE REGULARLY with SILVER MEDICAL, POLICE and FIRE COMMANDERS

➤ BRIEF all health service staff for duty on arrival
  • Delegate briefing of doctors and nurses to SILVER MEDICAL COMMANDER

➤ UPDATE ambulance GOLD regularly; pass information for hospitals through GOLD rather than direct to hospitals

➤ Consider how you will communicate with fixed points at the scene (for example, CCS, ambulance parking, ambulance loading): radio, mobile phone, field telephone, runner may be used
➤ Provide media brief when requested

  • Ensure any media briefings at scene are with knowledge of SILVER POLICE COMMANDER AND SILVER AMBULANCE COMMANDER

ASSESSMENT
➤ Identify areas for ambulance parking and CCS; establish an ambulance circuit (liaise with POLICE)
➤ Identify helicopter landing site and ensure is marked <<◆43-45◆>>
➤ Assess developing hazards to health service staff
➤ Assess need for additional ambulance and medical personnel and equipment resources; liaise with SILVER MEDICAL COMMANDER for number and type of medical resources
➤ Assess need to rest or relieve staff at scene

TRIAGE
➤ Ensure triage is being carried out at point of contact (primary triage) and at CCS (secondary triage); SECTORISE incident and appoint multiple primary triage officers; priorities for evacuation may differ from priorities for treatment at the scene <<◆30-36◆>>
➤ Determine the use of the EXPECTANT category, in conjunction with SILVER MEDICAL COMMANDER <<◆32◆>>

TREATMENT
➤ Establish a casualty clearing station; delegate running of CCS to doctor when available <<◆39◆>>
➤ Provide ambulance personnel to treat patients at point of first contact; bring forward medical personnel from CCS for specific tasks. Otherwise concentrate medical personnel at CCS
➤ Aim to achieve best practice standards, but accept compromise when resources are overwhelmed <<◆38◆>>

TRANSPORT
➤ Select appropriate transport for individual patients; liaise with LOADING OFFICER and SILVER MEDICAL COMMANDER to identify needs <<◆41-42◆>>

bronze ambulance commander

COMMAND
➤ Take orders from the SILVER AMBULANCE
COMMANDER
➤ Wear the tabard to identify yourself as the BRONZE
AMBULANCE COMMANDER
➤ Start a log of your actions, noting the time for each
entry; use a scribe when available

SAFETY
➤ Safety of all personnel inside the BRONZE area is
a responsibility of the BRONZE FIRE COMMANDER
➤ Staff may be tagged on entering BRONZE area,
when hazard is existent

COMMUNICATIONS
➤ LIAISE REGULARLY with BRONZE MEDICAL,
POLICE and FIRE COMMANDERS
➤ BRIEF all health service staff sent forward for
specific tasks
➤ UPDATE SILVER AMBULANCE COMMANDER
regularly
➤ Consider how you will communicate with SILVER
AMBULANCE COMMANDER, and other BRONZE
COMMANDERS: face-to-face, radio, mobile phone,
field telephone, runner may be used

ASSESSMENT
- ➤ Assess developing hazards to health service staff and liaise with BRONZE FIRE COMMANDER
- ➤ Assess need for additional ambulance and/or medical personnel and equipment resources; liaise with SILVER AMBULANCE COMMANDER for resources
- ➤ Assess need to rest or relieve staff at scene

TRIAGE
- ➤ Ensure triage is being carried out at point of contact (primary triage); SECTORISE incident and use multiple PRIMARY TRIAGE OFFICERS
- ➤ Implement the use of the EXPECTANT category at the discretion of SILVER AMBULANCE COMMANDER

TREATMENT
- ➤ Oversee CCS at discretion of SILVER AMBULANCE COMMANDER (not appropriate in all incidents); delegate running of CCS to doctor when available
- ➤ Direct ambulance personnel to treat patients at point of first contact; request medical and nursing personnel to come forward from CCS for specific tasks
- ➤ Aim to achieve best practice standards, but accept compromise when resources are overwhelmed

TRANSPORT
- ➤ Use available staff to transport patients to CCS: liaise with BRONZE FIRE COMMANDER and SILVER AMBULANCE COMMANDER for support

CCS officer

➤ Take orders from the SILVER AMBULANCE COMMANDER
➤ Wear the tabard to identify yourself as the CCS OFFICER
➤ Take command of CCS
➤ If not already done, select location:
  • hard standing where possible
  • close to vehicle circuit
  • safe distance from scene hazards
➤ Use existing or improvised shelter
➤ Clearly mark entrance to CCS and each priority area
➤ Assign staff to do triage: use SIEVE until adequate personnel to assist with SORT
➤ Place staff in a clinical area appropriate to their training and experience
➤ Orientate casualties with head towards the centre of a temporary shelter; do not overcrowd a shelter
➤ Set up equipment dump and delegate management of internal resupply to EQUIPMENT OFFICER
➤ Call forward vehicles as required for transport of casualties: liaise with PARKING OFFICER
➤ When CCS overwhelmed, do not attempt to treat P3 casualties at scene: transport with first aider/other medical assistance as escort
➤ Start to record destination of casualties treated in CCS and hand this responsibility to LOADING OFFICER
➤ Liaise with SILVER AMBULANCE COMMANDER for further staff and equipment resources
➤ Hand over responsibility of CCS to appointed DOCTOR

CCS layout

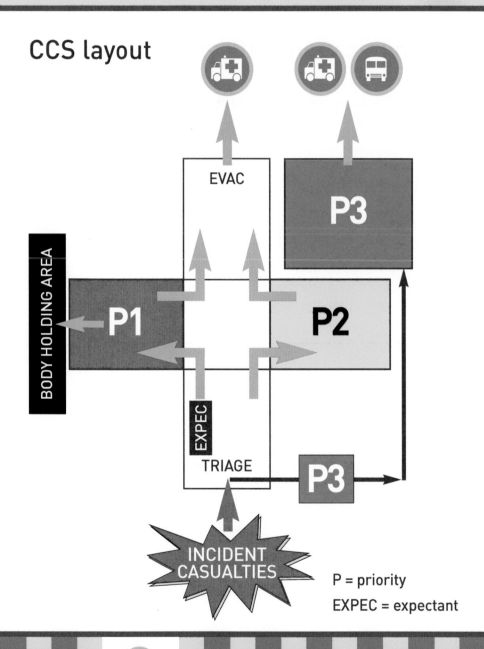

P = priority

EXPEC = expectant

communications officer

➤ Take orders from the SILVER AMBULANCE COMMANDER

➤ Work within the silver AMBULANCE COMMAND VEHICLE at scene

➤ Maintain a continuous message log, recording the time each message is received and the action taken

➤ Provide control for the health service radio net at the scene

➤ Issue radios, spare batteries and call-signs to appropriate health service staff at the scene

➤ Provide the communications link with GOLD ambulance command, and ensure GOLD is regularly updated

➤ Provide a communications link with hospitals directly or via GOLD ambulance command

METHANE report

M My call-sign, or name and appointment
Major incident STANDBY or DECLARED

E Exact location
- Grid reference, or GPS where available

T Type of incident

H Hazards, present and potential

A Access to scene, and egress route
- Helicopter landing site location

N Number and severity of casualties

E Emergency services, present and required

equipment officer

➤ Take orders from the SILVER AMBULANCE COMMANDER

➤ Wear the tabard to identify yourself as the EQUIPMENT OFFICER and work within the Casualty Clearing Station (CCS)

➤ Establish and maintain an equipment dump

➤ Receive requests for resupply of medical equipment, including oxygen and drugs, from CCS and bronze area
  - Provide resupply as individual items, or as exchange system for standardised rucksacks/equipment boxes
  - Ensure there is no duplication of supply for same patient, and that equipment reaches intended patient

➤ Forward requests for items required from off-site via silver ambulance command vehicle

➤ Inform SILVER AMBULANCE COMMANDER of critical equipment deficiencies

hierarchy of ambulance command

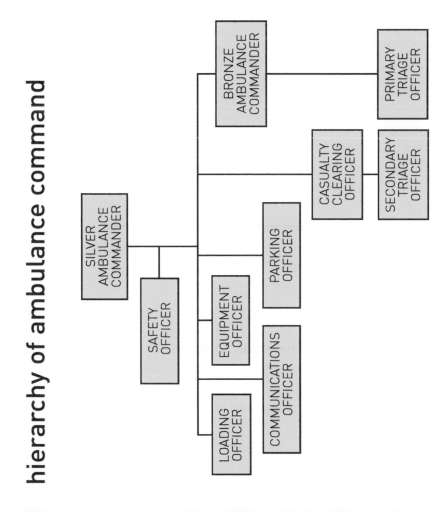

loading officer

- ➤ Take orders from the SILVER AMBULANCE COMMANDER
- ➤ Wear the tabard to identify yourself as the LOADING OFFICER
- ➤ Work within the CCS
- ➤ Establish a holding area for casualties awaiting evacuation. Ensure this area is adequately staffed and equipped (direct your personnel and equipment requirements to CCS COMMANDER)
- ➤ Supervise the triage of casualties for evacuation
- ➤ Select appropriate transport for individual casualties, liaising with a CCS doctor or SILVER AMBULANCE COMMANDER where necessary
- ➤ Liaise with PARKING OFFICER and call forward vehicles as required
- ➤ Evacuate casualties in priority order, allowing lesser priority casualties to be evacuated when packaging of higher priority casualties is incomplete
- ➤ Ensure patient packaging is adequate (secure lines; limb/spinal immobilisation; adequate fluids and analgesia)
- ➤ Ensure loading of helicopter(s) is supervised by trained staff
- ➤ Log destination of casualties

helicopter loading

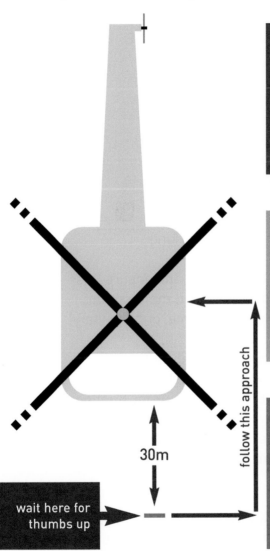

➤ Keep bystanders and animals clear
➤ Do not look towards the helicopter without eye protection
➤ Remove loose headgear

➤ Some small air ambulances will load through the tail
➤ Wait in front of aircraft for instructions from flight crew

➤ The danger area for TWIN ROTOR aircraft is at the front; remain >50m away and do not approach until instructed by ground staff

follow this approach

30m

wait here for thumbs up

parking officer

➤ Take orders from the SILVER AMBULANCE COMMANDER

➤ Wear the tabard to identify yourself as the PARKING OFFICER

➤ Establish a parking area for ambulance vehicles, ideally on hard standing and on/adjacent to vehicle circuit

➤ Co-ordinate ambulance vehicle parking

➤ Establish a helicopter landing site and ensure this is marked and manned by a trained marshal (this function may be undertaken by police, or by military)

➤ Receive ambulance crews and medical teams arriving by emergency vehicle: direct personnel to SILVER AMBULANCE COMMANDER for briefing

➤ Assess suitability of protective equipment of arriving staff and inform SAFETY OFFICER when clothing is inadequate

➤ Liaise with LOADING OFFICER for requirement to send vehicles forward to CCS for patient evacuation

helicopter landing site: selection

This is the recommended landing site preparation when the exact details of the aircraft are unknown

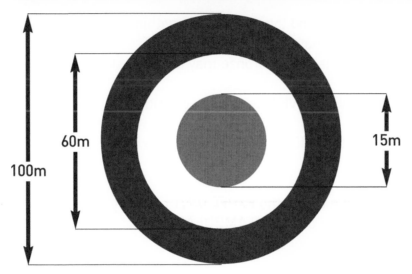

100m

60m

15m

1 metre = 1 pace

All areas must be cleared of loose objects

Ideally ground should be level: if sloping, slope should be uniform and <10°

Hard standing or firm ground capable of taking at least 4 tons

Cleared to ground level

Cleared to 0.6m (2 feet)

primary triage officer – 1

➤ Wear the tabard to identify yourself as the TRIAGE OFFICER

➤ Assign priorities and label casualties within the sector designated by the AMBULANCE COMMANDER (silver or bronze may assign task)

➤ Use the TRIAGE SIEVE (see over) to prioritise adults

➤ Use the PAEDIATRIC TRIAGE TAPE to prioritise children

➤ Implement the use of the EXPECTANT category at the discretion of SILVER AMBULANCE COMMANDER

➤ Keep a tally of the number of casualties of each priority within your assigned sector: report this to the AMBULANCE COMMANDER (BRONZE COMMANDER if appointed, otherwise SILVER COMMANDER)

➤ Once primary triage is complete accept further tasking from the SILVER AMBULANCE COMMANDER

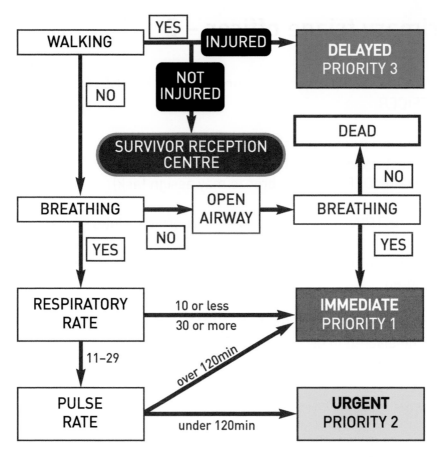

Capillary refill test (CRT) is an alternative to pulse rate, but is unreliable in the cold or dark: when used, a CRT >2 secs indicates PRIORITY 1

Keep a record of the NUMBER and PRIORITY of casualties you triage. Pass this to the AMBULANCE COMMANDER on completion

primary triage officer – 2

➤ Wear the tabard to identify yourself as the TRIAGE OFFICER

➤ Assign priorities and label casualties within the sector designated by the AMBULANCE COMMANDER (silver or bronze may assign task)

➤ Use the TRIAGE SIEVE (see over) to prioritise adults

➤ Use the PAEDIATRIC TRIAGE TAPE to prioritise children

➤ Implement the use of the EXPECTANT category at the discretion of SILVER AMBULANCE COMMANDER

➤ Keep a tally of the number of casualties of each priority within your assigned sector: report this to the AMBULANCE COMMANDER (BRONZE COMMANDER if appointed, otherwise SILVER COMMANDER)

➤ Once primary triage is complete accept further tasking from the SILVER AMBULANCE COMMANDER

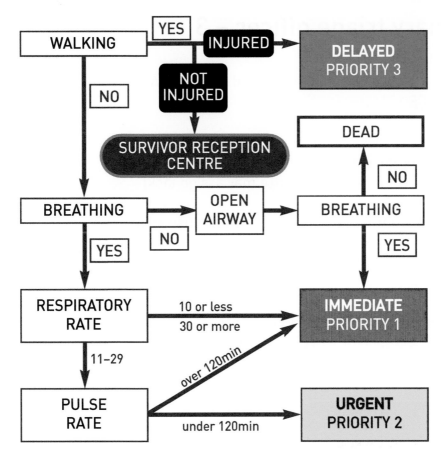

| WALKING | YES → INJURED → | DELAYED PRIORITY 3 |

- WALKING — YES → INJURED → **DELAYED** PRIORITY 3
- NOT INJURED → SURVIVOR RECEPTION CENTRE
- WALKING — NO ↓

BREATHING → NO → OPEN AIRWAY → BREATHING → NO → DEAD

BREATHING — YES ↓

RESPIRATORY RATE — 10 or less / 30 or more → **IMMEDIATE** PRIORITY 1

BREATHING → YES → **IMMEDIATE** PRIORITY 1

RESPIRATORY RATE — 11–29 ↓

PULSE RATE — over 120min → **IMMEDIATE** PRIORITY 1

PULSE RATE — under 120min → **URGENT** PRIORITY 2

Capillary refill test (CRT) is an alternative to pulse rate, but is unreliable in the cold or dark: when used, a CRT >2 secs indicates PRIORITY 1

Keep a record of the NUMBER and PRIORITY of casualties you triage. Pass this to the AMBULANCE COMMANDER on completion

primary triage officer – 3

➤ Wear the tabard to identify yourself as the TRIAGE OFFICER

➤ Assign priorities and label casualties within the sector designated by the AMBULANCE COMMANDER (silver or bronze may assign task)

➤ Use the TRIAGE SIEVE (see over) to prioritise adults

➤ Use the PAEDIATRIC TRIAGE TAPE to prioritise children

➤ Implement the use of the EXPECTANT category at the discretion of SILVER AMBULANCE COMMANDER

➤ Keep a tally of the number of casualties of each priority within your assigned sector: report this to the AMBULANCE COMMANDER (BRONZE COMMANDER if appointed, otherwise SILVER COMMANDER)

➤ Once primary triage is complete accept further tasking from the SILVER AMBULANCE COMMANDER

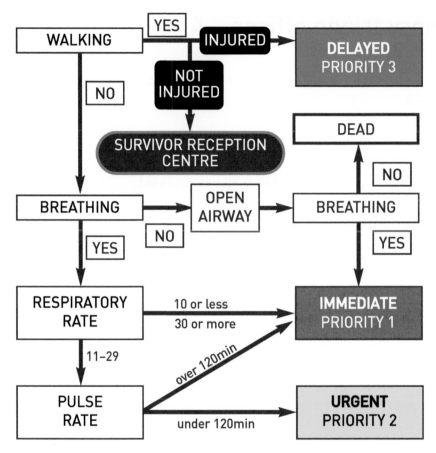

WALKING — **YES** → INJURED → **DELAYED** PRIORITY 3

NOT INJURED → SURVIVOR RECEPTION CENTRE

WALKING — NO → BREATHING

BREATHING — NO → OPEN AIRWAY → BREATHING

BREATHING — NO → DEAD

BREATHING — YES → IMMEDIATE PRIORITY 1

BREATHING — YES → RESPIRATORY RATE

RESPIRATORY RATE — 10 or less / 30 or more → **IMMEDIATE** PRIORITY 1

RESPIRATORY RATE — 11–29 → PULSE RATE

PULSE RATE — over 120min → **IMMEDIATE** PRIORITY 1

PULSE RATE — under 120min → **URGENT** PRIORITY 2

Capillary refill test (CRT) is an alternative to pulse rate, but is unreliable in the cold or dark: when used, a CRT >2 secs indicates PRIORITY 1

Keep a record of the NUMBER and PRIORITY of casualties you triage. Pass this to the AMBULANCE COMMANDER on completion

primary triage officer – 4

➤ Wear the tabard to identify yourself as the TRIAGE OFFICER

➤ Assign priorities and label casualties within the sector designated by the AMBULANCE COMMANDER (silver or bronze may assign task)

➤ Use the TRIAGE SIEVE (see over) to prioritise adults

➤ Use the PAEDIATRIC TRIAGE TAPE to prioritise children

➤ Implement the use of the EXPECTANT category at the discretion of SILVER AMBULANCE COMMANDER

➤ Keep a tally of the number of casualties of each priority within your assigned sector: report this to the AMBULANCE COMMANDER (BRONZE COMMANDER if appointed, otherwise SILVER COMMANDER)

➤ Once primary triage is complete accept further tasking from the SILVER AMBULANCE COMMANDER

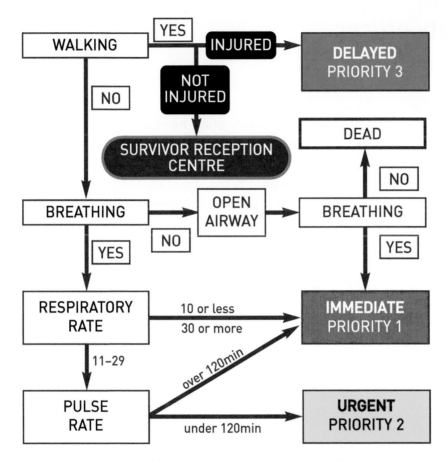

Capillary refill test (CRT) is an alternative to pulse rate, but is unreliable in the cold or dark: when used, a CRT >2 secs indicates PRIORITY 1

Keep a record of the NUMBER and PRIORITY of casualties you triage. Pass this to the AMBULANCE COMMANDER on completion

safety officer

- ➤ Wear the tabard to identify yourself as the SAFETY OFFICER
- ➤ Assume responsibility for the safety of all health service personnel at the scene
- ➤ Liaise with SILVER FIRE COMMANDER to identify existing or potential risks to health service staff, and inform SILVER AMBULANCE COMMANDER
- ➤ Ensure correct personal protective equipment (PPE) is worn by all health service personnel. Where correct PPE is not worn, refuse access to hazardous areas (staff are to be used in non-hazardous areas or are to be denied entry to the scene)
- ➤ It is a health service responsibility to ensure adequate decontamination of casualties. Where a specific chemical or radiation contamination risk exists, ensure that correct procedures are followed for protecting health service personnel and organising the decontamination of casualties (see over)
- ➤ Identify health service staff who require rest or replacement at the scene

decontamination

Casualty decontamination is a responsibility of the HEALTH SERVICES

The following procedure applies to decontamination from hazardous chemical, radiation or bio-hazard

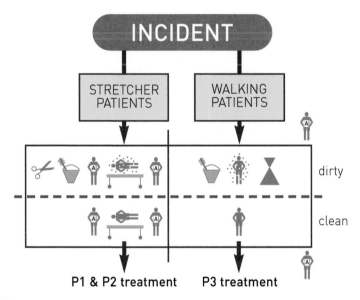

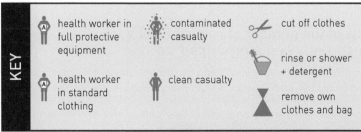

secondary triage officer

➤ Wear the tabard to identify yourself as the TRIAGE OFFICER

➤ Assign priorities to casualties on arrival at the casualty clearing station (casualties should already be labelled, but in some cases primary triage will have been missed)

➤ Use the TRIAGE SIEVE to prioritise adults when the casualty flow is high

➤ Use the TRIAGE SORT (see over) to prioritise adults when time and resources allow

➤ Use the PAEDIATRIC TRIAGE TAPE to prioritise all children

➤ Implement the use of the EXPECTANT category at the discretion of SILVER AMBULANCE COMMANDER

➤ Keep a tally of the number of casualties of each priority: report this to the CCS OFFICER

STEP 1: calculate the GLASGOW COMA SCORE (GCS)

A Eye opening:	
spontaneous	4
to voice	3
to pain	2
none	1

B Verbal response:	
orientated	5
confused	4
inappropriate	3
incomprehensible	2
no response	1

C Motor response:	
obeys commands	6
localises	5
pain withdraws	4
pain flexes	3
pain extends	2
no response	1

GCS= A + B + C

STEP 2: calculate the TRIAGE SORT SCORE

X GCS		Y Respiratory rate		Z Systolic BP	
13-15	4	10-29	4	90 or more	4
9-12	3	30 or more	3	76-89	3
6-8	2	6-9	2	50-75	2
4-5	1	1-5	1	1-49	1
3	0	0	0	0	0

TRIAGE SORT SCORE = X + Y + Z

STEP 3: assign a triage PRIORITY

> **12 = PRIORITY 3**
> **11 = PRIORITY 2**
> **<10 = PRIORITY 1**

STEP 4: upgrade PRIORITY at discretion of senior clinician, dependent on the anatomical injury/working diagnosis

> Keep a record of the NUMBER and PRIORITY of casualties you triage. Pass this to the AMBULANCE COMMANDER on completion

ACTION CARDS
medical personnel

11	silver medical commander
12	bronze medical commander
13	Casualty Clearing Station commander
14	secondary triage officer
15	medical team leader
16	body holding area doctor

action card ➤ ➤ ➤ ➤ ➤ ➤ ➤ **11**

silver medical commander

COMMAND

- ➤ Take COMMAND of all medical and nursing assets; make key appointments
- ➤ Wear the tabard to identify yourself as the SILVER MEDICAL COMMANDER. Remain near SILVER AMBULANCE COMMANDER as much as possible
- ➤ Precedence for command rests with SILVER AMBULANCE COMMANDER
- ➤ Start a log of your actions, noting the time for each entry; use a scribe when available

SAFETY

- ➤ Take responsibility for the safety of doctors and nurses at scene, or more usually is delegated to SAFETY OFFICER (action card 9)

COMMUNICATIONS

- ➤ LIAISE REGULARLY with SILVER POLICE and FIRE COMMANDERS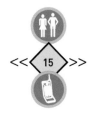
- ➤ BRIEF doctors and nurses for duty
- ➤ Information for hospitals is best passed through ambulance GOLD rather than direct
- ➤ Consider how you will communicate with fixed points at the scene (for example, CCS): radio, mobile phone, field telephone or runner may be used
- ➤ Provide media brief when requested
  - Ensure any media briefings at scene are with knowledge of SILVER POLICE COMMANDER

ASSESSMENT

➤ Reassess location and layout of CCS; reconfigure if necessary

➤ Assess need for additional medical personnel and equipment resources; communicate this to SILVER AMBULANCE COMMANDER

➤ Assess need to rest or relieve staff at scene

➤ Provide staff to assist with triage at point of first contact or at CCS, in liaison with SILVER AMBULANCE COMMANDER

➤ Allow senior clinicians to use judgment to adjust physiological triage priorities based on anatomy of injury or clinical diagnosis

➤ Determine the use of the EXPECTANT category, in conjunction with silver ambulance commander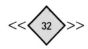

TREATMENT

➤ Establish a casualty clearing station if not already done; appoint a doctor to run CCS when available

➤ Provide medical and nursing personnel from CCS to move forward for specific tasks. Otherwise concentrate medical personnel at CCS

➤ Aim to achieve best practice standards, but accept compromise when resources are overwhelmed

TRANSPORT

➤ Liaise with SILVER AMBULANCE COMMANDER to identify specific transport needs for individual patients

➤ Provide nursing or medical escorts for individual patients where necessary

<< DOC >>

bronze medical commander

COMMAND
- ➤ Take orders from the SILVER MEDICAL COMMANDER
- ➤ Wear the tabard to identify yourself as the BRONZE MEDICAL COMMANDER
- ➤ Start a log of your actions, noting the time for each entry; use a scribe when available

SAFETY
- ➤ Safety of all personnel inside the bronze area is a responsibility of the BRONZE FIRE COMMANDER
- ➤ Staff may be tagged on entering BRONZE area, when hazard is existent

COMMUNICATIONS
- ➤ LIAISE REGULARLY with BRONZE AMBULANCE, POLICE and FIRE commanders
- ➤ BRIEF all medical and nursing staff sent forward for specific tasks
- ➤ UPDATE SILVER MEDICAL COMMANDER regularly
- ➤ Consider how you will communicate with SILVER MEDICAL COMMANDER, and other BRONZE COMMANDERS: face-to-face, radio, mobile phone, field telephone or runner may be used

ASSESSMENT
- ➤ Assess need for additional medical and/or nursing personnel and equipment resources; liaise with SILVER MEDICAL COMMANDER for resources
- ➤ Assess need to rest or relieve staff at scene

TRIAGE
- ➤ Provide staff to assist with triage at point of first contact, in liaison with SILVER MEDICAL COMMANDER
- ➤ Allow senior clinicians to use judgment to adjust physiological triage priorities based on anatomy of injury or clinical diagnosis
- ➤ Implement the use of the EXPECTANT category at the discretion of SILVER MEDICAL COMMANDER

TREATMENT
- ➤ Oversee CCS at discretion of SILVER MEDICAL COMMANDER (not appropriate in all incidents); delegate running of CCS to doctor when available
- ➤ Direct medical and nursing personnel to treat patients at point of first contact when called forward from CCS for specific tasks
- ➤ Aim to achieve best practice standards, but accept compromise when resources are overwhelmed

TRANSPORT
- ➤ Provide appropriate escort of nurse or doctor to CCS with individual patients (if team called forward to treat patient, it should return to CCS with patient)

CCS commander

➤ Receive briefing from SILVER MEDICAL COMMANDER
➤ Wear tabard to identify yourself as CCS COMMANDER
➤ If not already done, select location:
  • Hard standing where possible
  • Close to vehicle circuit
  • Safe distance from scene hazards
➤ Use existing or improvised shelter
➤ Clearly mark entrance to CCS and priority areas
➤ Assign staff to triage: use SIEVE until adequate personnel to assist with SORT
➤ Place staff in clinical area appropriate to training and experience
➤ Orientate casualties with head towards centre of temporary shelter, and do not overcrowd shelter
➤ Set up equipment dump and delegate management of internal resupply to EQUIPMENT OFFICER
➤ Call forward vehicles as required for transport of casualties: liaise with PARKING OFFICER
➤ When CCS overwhelmed, do not attempt to treat P3 casualties at scene: transport with first aider/other medical assistance as escort
➤ Start to record destination of casualties treated in CCS and hand this responsibility to LOADING OFFICER
➤ Liaise with SILVER AMBULANCE COMMANDER for further staff and equipment resources
➤ Hand over responsibility of CCS to appointed DOCTOR

CCS layout

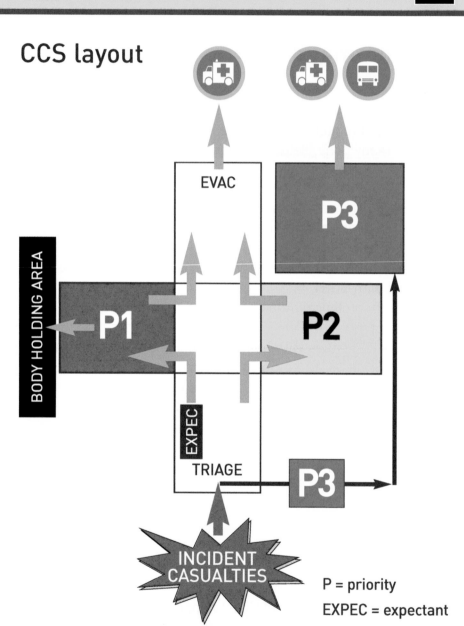

P = priority

EXPEC = expectant

secondary triage officer

➤ Wear the tabard to identify yourself as the TRIAGE
OFFICER

➤ Assign priorities to casualties on arrival at the
Casualty Clearing Station (casualties should
already be labelled, but in some cases primary
triage will have been missed)

➤ Use the TRIAGE SIEVE to prioritise adults when the
casualty flow is high

➤ Use the TRIAGE SORT (see over) to prioritise adults
when time and resources allow

➤ Use the PAEDIATRIC TRIAGE TAPE to prioritise
all children

➤ Allow senior clinicians to use judgement to adjust
physiological triage priorities based on anatomy
of injury or clinical diagnosis

➤ Implement the use of the EXPECTANT category
at the discretion of SILVER MEDICAL COMMANDER

➤ Keep a tally of the number of casualties of each
priority: report this to the CCS COMMANDER

STEP 1: calculate the GLASGOW COMA SCORE (GCS)

A Eye opening:	
spontaneous	4
to voice	3
to pain	2
none	1

B Verbal response:	
orientated	5
confused	4
inappropriate	3
incomprehensible	2
no response	1

C Motor response:	
obeys commands	6
localises	5
pain withdraws	4
pain flexes	3
pain extends	2
no response	1

GCS= A + B + C

STEP 2: calculate the TRIAGE SORT SCORE

X GCS	
13-15	4
9-12	3
6-8	2
4-5	1
3	0

Y Respiratory rate	
10-29	4
30 or more	3
6-9	2
1-5	1
0	0

Z Systolic BP	
90 or more	4
76-89	3
50-75	2
1-49	1
0	0

TRIAGE SORT SCORE = X + Y + Z

STEP 3: assign a triage PRIORITY

12	=	PRIORITY 3
11	=	PRIORITY 2
<10	=	PRIORITY 1

STEP 4: upgrade PRIORITY at discretion of senior clinician, dependent on the anatomical injury/working diagnosis

Keep a record of the NUMBER and PRIORITY of casualties you triage. Pass this to the AMBULANCE COMMANDER on completion

<< DOC >>

medical team leader – 1

- ➤ Receive briefing from SILVER MEDICAL COMMANDER

- ➤ Work in CCS under direction of CCS COMMANDER

- ➤ Distribute medical equipment brought with team according to CCS COMMANDER (may be required to leave in equipment dump)

- ➤ Move forward as whole or part of team for specific task

- ➤ Confirm with BRONZE MEDICAL/AMBULANCE COMMANDER on completion of task that return to CCS, or remain on site for supplementary task

- ➤ Monitor welfare of team, and appropriate use of staff according to skills

- ➤ Communicate with CCS COMMANDER need for resupply of medical equipment, and need for further medical support

- ➤ Act as escorts for critical patients as deemed appropriate by CCS COMMANDER or SILVER MEDICAL COMMANDER

treatment priorities

Treatment priorities for individual patients follow best practice within the constraints of a multiple casualty incident:

AIRWAY, with cervical spine control where appropriate
BREATHING, with oxygen where available
CIRCULATION, with control of external bleeding always

Major incident treatment limitations

➤ Full *spinal immobilisation* is impractical for all victims of, for example, a rail crash, even though they are exposed to the same mechanism of injury. Clinical judgement must be exercised to a greater extent than in a single casualty blunt trauma incident

➤ *Oxygen* is a limited resource: more than one patient can be given oxygen from the same cylinder (use a Y connector), but individual flow rates may be reduced

➤ *Defibrillation* may be appropriate in the casualty clearing station for a witnessed cardiac arrest: those with no vital signs at the site of injury should be declared dead

➤ *Intubation* can only be performed by paramedics on unresponsive (dead or nearly dead) patients: it has a limited role at the scene

medical team leader – 2

➤ Receive briefing from SILVER MEDICAL COMMANDER

➤ Work in CCS under direction of CCS COMMANDER

➤ Distribute medical equipment brought with team according to CCS COMMANDER (may be required to leave in equipment dump)

➤ Move forward as whole or part of team for specific task

➤ Confirm with BRONZE MEDICAL/AMBULANCE COMMANDER on completion of task that return to CCS, or remain on site for supplementary task

➤ Monitor welfare of team, and appropriate use of staff according to skills

➤ Communicate with CCS COMMANDER need for resupply of medical equipment, and need for further medical support

➤ Act as escorts for critical patients as deemed appropriate by CCS COMMANDER or SILVER MEDICAL COMMANDER

treatment priorities

Treatment priorities for individual patients follow best practice within the constraints of a multiple casualty incident:

AIRWAY, with cervical spine control where appropriate
BREATHING, with oxygen where available
CIRCULATION, with control of external bleeding always

Major incident treatment limitations

➤ Full *spinal immobilisation* is impractical for all victims of, for example, a rail crash, even though they are exposed to the same mechanism of injury. Clinical judgement must be exercised to a greater extent than in a single casualty blunt trauma incident

➤ *Oxygen* is a limited resource: more than one patient can be given oxygen from the same cylinder (use a Y connector), but individual flow rates may be reduced

➤ *Defibrillation* may be appropriate in the casualty clearing station for a witnessed cardiac arrest: those with no vital signs at the site of injury should be declared dead

➤ *Intubation* can only be performed by paramedics on unresponsive (dead or nearly dead) patients: it has a limited role at the scene

medical team leader – 3

➤ Receive briefing from SILVER MEDICAL COMMANDER

➤ Work in CCS under direction of CCS COMMANDER

➤ Distribute medical equipment brought with team according to CCS COMMANDER (may be required to leave in equipment dump)

➤ Move forward as whole or part of team for specific task

➤ Confirm with BRONZE MEDICAL/AMBULANCE COMMANDER on completion of task that return to CCS, or remain on site for supplementary task

➤ Monitor welfare of team, and appropriate use of staff according to skills

➤ Communicate with CCS COMMANDER need for resupply of medical equipment, and need for further medical support

➤ Act as escorts for critical patients as deemed appropriate by CCS COMMANDER or SILVER MEDICAL COMMANDER

treatment priorities

Treatment priorities for individual patients follow best practice within the constraints of a multiple casualty incident:

AIRWAY, with cervical spine control where appropriate
BREATHING, with oxygen where available
CIRCULATION, with control of external bleeding always

Major incident treatment limitations

➤ Full *spinal immobilisation* is impractical for all victims of, for example, a rail crash, even though they are exposed to the same mechanism of injury. Clinical judgement must be exercised to a greater extent than in a single casualty blunt trauma incident

➤ *Oxygen* is a limited resource: more than one patient can be given oxygen from the same cylinder (use a Y connector), but individual flow rates may be reduced

➤ *Defibrillation* may be appropriate in the casualty clearing station for a witnessed cardiac arrest: those with no vital signs at the site of injury should be declared dead

➤ *Intubation* can only be performed by paramedics on unresponsive (dead or nearly dead) patients: it has a limited role at the scene

medical team leader – 4

➤ Receive briefing from SILVER MEDICAL COMMANDER

➤ Work in CCS under direction of CCS COMMANDER

➤ Distribute medical equipment brought with team according to CCS COMMANDER (may be required to leave in equipment dump)

➤ Move forward as whole or part of team for specific task

➤ Confirm with BRONZE MEDICAL/AMBULANCE COMMANDER on completion of task that return to CCS, or remain on site for supplementary task

➤ Monitor welfare of team, and appropriate use of staff according to skills

➤ Communicate with CCS COMMANDER need for resupply of medical equipment, and need for further medical support

➤ Act as escorts for critical patients as deemed appropriate by CCS COMMANDER or SILVER MEDICAL COMMANDER

treatment priorities

Treatment priorities for individual patients follow best practice within the constraints of a multiple casualty incident:

AIRWAY, with cervical spine control where appropriate
BREATHING, with oxygen where available
CIRCULATION, with control of external bleeding always

Major incident treatment limitations

➤ Full *spinal immobilisation* is impractical for all victims of, for example, a rail crash, even though they are exposed to the same mechanism of injury. Clinical judgement must be exercised to a greater extent than in a single casualty blunt trauma incident

➤ *Oxygen* is a limited resource: more than one patient can be given oxygen from the same cylinder (use a Y connector), but individual flow rates may be reduced

➤ *Defibrillation* may be appropriate in the casualty clearing station for a witnessed cardiac arrest: those with no vital signs at the site of injury should be declared dead

➤ *Intubation* can only be performed by paramedics on unresponsive (dead or nearly dead) patients: it has a limited role at the scene

body holding area doctor

➤ Receive briefing from SILVER MEDICAL COMMANDER

➤ Work in CCS under direction of CCS COMMANDER

➤ Pronounce death in presence of police officer and record:
- date and time
- your name
- police officer's name/number

➤ Move forward onto incident at direction of SILVER MEDICAL COMMANDER to assist police with pronouncing death at point of injury

> ➤ NOTE:
> - Death is **DIAGNOSED** by any individual trained to use a triage protocol and apply a triage label
> - Death is **PRONOUNCED** by a doctor at the scene, in the presence of a police officer
> - Death is **CERTIFIED** by the pathologist performing the post-mortem examination

hierarchy of medical command

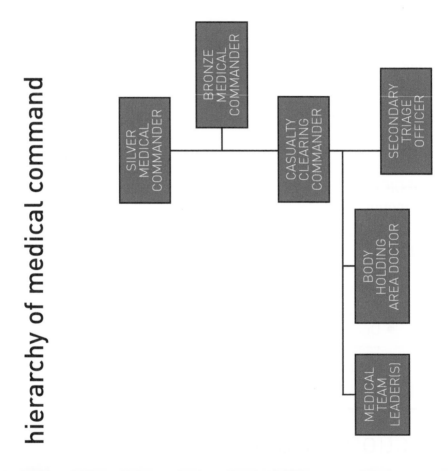

INCIDENT LOG

Printed and bound by CPI Group (UK) Ltd, Croydon, CR0 4YY
25/07/2022
03138025-0001